Food Regeneration Guide Blood Group B

ISBN 978-1-312-25875-4

MANUEL RAMONI... NEURO-THERAPIST

Worse Foods (*Blood Bundles, Sick and Aged*). ___Wheat, Corn, Pork, Chicken, Delicatessen, Avocado, Tomato, Fried Meals, Shrimp, Peanuts, White Sugar___

FOOD ACCORDING TO YOUR BLOOD GROUP.
BLOOD GROUP "B" - THE SHEPHERD.

What you will learn in the following pages will change your life and that of your loved ones forever and in such a precise and safe way that in a few weeks they will feel the changes in their body in such a radical and different way, that They will feel and will be younger, stronger, more vigorous, full of energy, vitality and most importantly ... Full of great **health and that when any viral or bacterial disease wants to enter their body, they will hardly feel a breakdown since** their immune system and "**ALKALINITY**" (This I will show you later) will be so strong that it will be almost impossible for them to ever get sick again (this if they keep their new culture of eating and living that I will teach them for life) and consequently take them to live the 100-year-old average.

Dr. Peter D`adamo, a deeply scientific researcher and pioneer in the field of food according to blood groups, has managed to compile through many scientific studies in different cultures and around many countries in the world. The way and way of classifying food according to the type of blood of human beings.

He managed to bring as much food as possible to the laboratory on his tour around the world and took each food and looked at it through the microscope with a blood sample of the different types that there are (4), type "O" - "A" - "B" and "AB" and managed to observe very carefully what was happening.

He managed to see that by placing the different types of food in the different types of blood, that these presented totally different characteristics from each other, that is; A) That there was a group of foods that made the blood more fluid, light and thin. B) A second group made absolutely no changes to it. C) While a third group surprisingly had clumping of the blood, that is, it made it thick and even coagulated.

So I manage to divide the food very intelligently and amazingly into three groups.

1- The foods that make the blood more fluid and less viscous or thick, making it feed (Carrying oxygen) in a very important way to all the cells of the body, passing through the thinnest capillaries of the body, nourishing, regenerating them and rejuvenating cell tissue in an extremely vital way for the body. As well as at the same time making the minute volume of the heart the most suitable for the body, thus reducing the overload that the heart needs when the blood is thick and very intoxicated... And he called them **VERY BENEFICIAL FOODS.**

2- A second group of foods that did not present or give any change in blood behavior that called them **NEUTRAL FOODS.**

3- And a third group of foods in which he noticed that in a very important way they presented clumping of the blood, making it more viscous and thick and thus hindering its function to the point that it was the main cause of premature cellular aging and called: **HARMFUL FOODS, NOT ADVISABLE OR "POISON" FOOD.** Therefore it determined after deep studies that each blood group has its indispensable food pattern and different from each other, that is, the foods that can be beneficial for a certain blood group... It is totally harmful to others.

1) **VERY BENEFICIAL:** Rejuvenate, Slim, Regenerate, Regulate Cardiac Minute Volume And Extend Life.

2) **NEUTRAL: They** feed but do not regenerate, nor do anything that group 1 does.

3) **NOT ADVISABLE:** They fatten, agglutinate (Thicken) the blood, poison the body, overload the heart, age and degenerate the cellular system.

Below I am going to expose you after many years of study and research on my part, as I have managed to summarize in broad terms the foods according to each blood group.

This I achieved thanks to GOD in tens of thousands of patients that I have seen in more than 39 years of consultation and follow-up, which with a lot of work and diligence I carried out in the deep study of each food in each blood group. Therefore, each region, country and its customs are of utmost importance.

For example, in the case of Venezuela there is the custom of the so-called pre-cooked flour or "bread flour", which has been consumed in large proportions in Venezuelan households for more than 66 years, and I realized that the sub generations following the continuous consumption of certain foods that are in principle of the group of harmful, the body adapts to the same for living and converts food HARMFUL food NEUTROS, with low toxicity, depending on the degree of generations that have crossed.

Other examples would be: Mexico, Chile (Spicy), Panamá, The Fritters, Brazil, La Feijoada (Black beans), Colombia the potatoes, Spain, Wine, etc.

Another thing that I learned unequivocally through so many years of monitoring, practice and study, is that; There are industrialized "foods" on the market that they sell to consumers in order to lose weight by substituting some of the main meals for a shake, which among other things, poorly combining, refined and industrialized carbohydrates with processed proteins (highly harmful combination, (Which we will talk about on the alkalinity life - acidification and death) In the Complete Guide to Healthy Longevity ...

That it "loses weight" but "dries" them at the same time, since the loss of collagen is progressive, and worst of all is that after the patient having spent fortunes on these "foods" they gain weight again unless they follow the diet regimen. "Products", something that will never happen with The Aliments According to its Blood Group.

There are basically three different types of protein shakes depending on the source from which those proteins are obtained, which may well be from whey (Poison for group O), egg white or soy (Poison for other groups) . The consumer does not have the slightest idea of how their body is poisoned (Acidifying it) with these drinks that keep them "full" but that far from nourishing the immune system, what is sinking it in an ending that always ends up leading to the query.

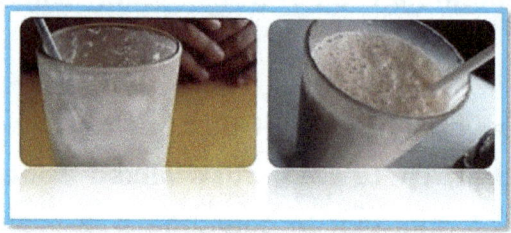

Scientific researchers at the University of California, San Francisco studied 9,000 women and found that those who consumed these products were about four times more likely to have hip fractures, among other things, than those who did not consume these "foods."

An unbalanced diet (Since it is the same "food" for everyone equally... "And no one is the same as another", especially in your blood group) "high in proteins, such as those from shakes, will directly contribute to having fragile bones or osteoporosis among other serious conditions that you will have in the medium or short term, more likely in some than others, depending on your vitality and blood group.

"Eating these artificial and highly harmful" foods "is like smoking and saying ... "It doesn't hurt me"

Keep in mind that according to the different food cultures that I will indicate for each blood group in particular, there are also people who are "secretory" and "non-secretory".

SECRETORS. A person is secretory, regardless of their blood group. It is when the antigens of your blood group are present both in your blood and in your body fluids and secretions, such as saliva, intestinal mucus or respiratory cavities, semen, etc.

NO SECRETARIES. A non-secretor, it does not secrete antigen from its group in its fluids but only in its blood.

Many metabolic characteristics such as carbohydrate intolerance or immune susceptibilities are genetically linked to the non-secretory subtype. A certain disadvantage is supposed compared to the "secretors", since these, when secreting the antigen from their blood group in their saliva and the intestinal mucus, have "extra" protection against certain microorganisms and lectins of some foods.

Another additional advantage of secretors is that they are able to maintain a more stable ecosystem of bifid intestinal bacteria suitable for their group. Most of these bifid bacteria use their blood group as the preferred food source, and since secretors have a higher blood volume in the intestinal mucus, their bacteria benefit from a more constant supply of food.

Approximately 80% of the world population are "secretaries". While 20% are Non-Secretaries. Therefore, it is important to repeat that the following list of foods according to your blood group has been adapted to correct these disagreements when shopping at the supermarket. And something of which I will be very emphatic... DO NOT PUT ANY FOOD OUT OF YOUR BLOOD GROUP IN THE CART WHEN MAKING THE MARKET for you.

With this new culture of eating, you will be able to eat whatever you want and as many times as you want to eat, as long as it is in the range of foods indicated according to your blood group, such as those that are advisable and neutral, but never the "poisons". You will not only lose weight quickly and progressively, but a date will come when you will not lose weight anymore since at that moment you will have reached your ideal natural weight and can continue eating as many times as you want during the day and **NOT** You will never gain more weight in your life and if you are a thin person, then not only will you feel better, but you will soon be in your necessary size and according to your age, but with a full immune system on top and prepared to fight any attack exogenous...

It is for this and other reasons that you will see in the course of the content of this Guide that I have successfully managed to eradicate diseases from a sick body and cure patients ranging from simple obesity to cancer of any kind and thanks to *GOD*. In more than 45 years of experience and unless it is due to natural causes, I HAVE NEVER LOST A PATIENT...

BLOOD GROUP "B" - THE SHEPHERD.

It is balanced. **He has a powerful immune system and a tolerant digestive system,** has more flexible food options and is a **consumer of dairy products.** Respond better to stress with creativity and requires a balance of physical and mental activity to stay slim and spirited.

It is the quintessential survivor and **least vulnerable** to many of the common diseases in other blood groups such as **heart conditions and cancer.** Even if you do contract them, you are more likely to survive them, but you are more prone to exotic immune system disorders like **multiple sclerosis, lupus, and chronic fatigue syndrome.** A high number of Asians and the majority of Jews (regardless of their geographical location) are **type B.**

Foods that **contribute to cell degeneration and weight gain are: corn, buckwheat, lentils, peanuts, and sesame seeds** that, although they have a different lectin, all affect the efficiency of their metabolic process **causing fatigue, fluid retention and hypoglycemia.**

Certain foods cause a reaction in blood sugar, especially those in group B. **The gluten lectin found in wheat germ and Wholemeal flour products slows your metabolism and is stored as fat.**

Foods that contribute to cell regeneration and weight loss are green leafy vegetables, allowed

meat, eggs, dairy products, and liver (they promote metabolic efficiency).

Soy foods can be eaten, but should not be used as a substitute for the **meat allowed for this group, as well as the fish and dairy that type B needs for optimal health.**

People in this group B diabetic who want to lose their weight and volume have to suspend, beers, flours and carbohydrates during the treatment to lose weight, whether they are Very **Beneficial** or Neutral. Because they interfere with the purification of the body. And after they have finished the weight loss period and are at their ideal weight they can eat these foods as long as they are in the allowed foods.

This group emerged about 10-15,000 years ago with the development of grazing. Their diet often consisted of milk and dairy products, with which after thousands of years their metabolism is more adapted to digest these foods.

- **Balanced.**
- **Powerful immune system.**
- **Tolerant digestive system.**
- **More flexible food options.**
- **Consumer of dairy products.**
- **Responds better to stress with creativity.**
- **Requires a balance between physical and mental activity to stay lean and spirited.**

- Blood group "B" developed 10,000 years ago after the introduction of grains into human nutrition.
- Those in this group can digest a wide variety of foods, including dairy and fermented products.
- Those in group "B" tend to be creative and unconventional.
- Type "B" is found in 10% of Caucasians and 20% of blacks.

Next I will indicate the list of foods for the group "B" **updated** and compiled with studies of many years of strategic follow-up for each blood group. That will make them lose overweight and diseases of any kind of which they are possessors with knowledge or that these diseases are in you in full development and you still do not know it.

PEOPLE WHO WANT TO LOWER THEIR WEIGHT AND VOLUME.

They have to suspend, sweets**, beers, flours and all carbohydrates** during the treatment to lose weight, whether they are Very **Beneficial** or Neutral. Because they interfere with the purification of the body. And after they have reached their ideal weight they will be able to eat these foods as long as they are in the beneficial foods.

Next I will indicate the list of foods for group B updated and compiled with studies of many years of strategic follow-up for each blood group. That will make them lose overweight and diseases of any kind of which they are possessors with knowledge or that these diseases are in full development and you do not know it yet.

It is of utmost importance due to the change of name of foods according to the region, the country or the culture; that when they get the name of a food in the lists that I indicate below and they do not know it. **Search the Internet with the name of the food and its synonym.** Then with **the name of the food in question, look** in the part of **Google images** and thus you can recognize the food.

Formula for "B":

It is imperative to do the three main meals and the three snacks since your metabolism is highly energy consuming to keep mental activity in harmony ... You should never miss out on your snacks (in addition to what you want to eat within your allowed meals) green tea , cheese and salads with cheese.

Beneficial Meats, Fish.	20%
Neutral Meats, Fish.	20%
Beneficial vegetables, dairy, eggs and oils.	25%
Neutral Vegetables.	10%
Beneficial Tea.	10%
Beneficial or Neutral Carbs.	10%
Rest of Beneficial and Neutral Foods.	10%

MEATS.

Very Beneficial: Goat, Lamb (sheep, goat, goat), Ram (sheep, sheep), Rabbit, Deer.

Neutrals: Ostrich, Buffalo, Beef, Smoked Meat (Beef), Salted Meat, Pheasant, Beef Liver, Turkey, Veal (Beef).

Not Recommended: Squirrel, Horse, Pig, Quail, Heart, Hen, Goose, Ham, Pigeon, Duck, Partridge, Chicken, Bacon, Turtle. Do not eat charcuterie, nor fried foods.

FISH AND SEAFOOD.

Avoid all shellfish, crab, lobster, shrimp, etc. Because they contain lectins that dangerously interfere with your system.

Very Beneficial: Cod, Sea bream (mojarra), Mackerel (bonito), Caviar, Dolphin, Haddock, Sturgeon, Hypoglossal, Horse mackerel, Sole, Pike, Hake, Grouper, Meerbrasse, Pompano (palometa), Oceanic Perch, Monkfish, Monkfish, Turbot, Tarpon, Salmon, Red mullet (threshing or barbel), Sardine.

Neutrals : Abalones (abalones), Fresh herring, Tuna, Blue whiting, Catfish, Calpa, Squid, Carite, Carp, Catalan, Cataco, Dogfish, Corigono, Corocoro, Corvina, Cubera, Red Cubera, Dorado, Smelt, Múgil, Snapper Red and White, Swordfish, Catfish, Parrotfish, Sunfish, Sailfish, Flounder, Shark, Sea Trout.

Not Recommended: Pollock, Clam, Anchovy, Frog Legs, Eel, Barracuda, Beluga, Lobster, Shrimp, Crab, Snails, White Sturgeon, Prawns, Salmon Eggs, Lobster, Prawn, Sea Bass, Amberjack, Mussel, Mollusks, Oysters, River Perch, Sunfish, Octopus, Frogs, Snook, Smoked Salmon, Turtle, Freshwater Trout of any kind, Scallops.

EGGS AND MILK.

You can enjoy the variety of dairy foods because the main sugar in the B antigen is Dgalactosamine present in milk as well. Start by introducing dairy starting with fermented or cultured ones like yogurt **and kefir** that are better tolerated than ice cream, whole milk, and cream cheese.

Very Beneficial: Whey Milk, Cow's Milk of all kinds, Goat's Milk, Cottage Cheese, Sheep Cheese (feta), Mozzarella Cheese, Goat Cheese, Fermerkase Ranchero Cheese, Kefir (fermented goat's milk), Paneer (fresh cheese from India), Ricotta, Yogurt.

Neutrals: Eggs 3 to 4 weekly (chicken or hen only), Curd, Sour Cream, Almond Milk, Brie Cheese, Ball Cheese, Gouda Cheese, Colby Cheese, Gruyere Cheese, Cream Cheese, Fresh Cheese, Hüttenkäse (German) , Jarlsburg Cheese, Crineja Cheese, Telita Cheese, Emmenthal Cheese, Hand Cheese, Llanero Cheese, Camembert Cheese, Edam Cheese, Munster Cheese, Casein Cheese, Cheddar Cheese, Neufchatel Cheese, Cream-Based Ice Cream (ask before to eat them, there are ice creams that are based on butter), Almond Milk, Whole Milk, Animal Butter, Nut Margarine, Buttermilk .

Not Advisable: Goose, Duck and Quail Eggs, Coconut Milk, Soy Milk, Soy Cheese, Blue Cheese, American Cheese (Cheddar type), Processed Cheese, Parmesan Cheese, Provolone Cheese, Roquefort Cheese, Peanut Margarine.

OILS.

Very Beneficial: Olive Oil, Linseed Oil (flax seed), Blackcurrant Oil, Walnut Oil. (For proper digestion and healthy bowel movements).

Neutrals: Coconut Oil (little), Cod Liver Oil, Almond Oil, Wheat Germ Oil, Evening Primrose Oil, Butter (animal).

Not Recommended: Canola Oil, Safflower Oil, Borage Oil, Corn Oil, Sunflower Oil, Peanut Oil, Rapeseed Oil, Castor Oil, Castor Oil, Sesame Oil, Cotton Oil, Soybean Oil.

DRY FRUITS AND SEEDS.

Most are not advised because they interfere with insulin production.

The fruits can then be eaten moderately.

Neutrals: Almonds, Cocoa, Chestnuts, Mushrooms, Beechnuts, Almond Margarine, Walnut, Pará Nut, Nefelio Nut, Pecan Nut, Flax Seeds.

Not Advisable: Hazelnuts, Sunflower, Peanut, Sunflower Margarine, Sunflower Seeds, Peanut Margarine, Sesame (tahini), Cashew Nuts (merey), Pine Nuts, Pistachio, Poppy Seeds, Pumpkin Seeds, Safflower Seeds, Sesame seeds.

VEGETABLES.

You should limit your intake to the **Very Beneficial** and eat them **very sporadically**.

Very Beneficial: Beans, Coffee, Soy Germ, Half Moon Bean.

Neutrals: Peas, Pods, Beans, Green Beans, beans, White Beans, Red Beans, Jícama Beans and Tamarind.

Not Advisable: Chickpeas, Red and Green Lentils, Green Beans, Beans and Speckled Beans, Soy Products, Tempe (tofu).

CEREALS.

Wheat is not well tolerated by most group B because it contains a lectin that attacks the insulin receptors of adipose tissue cells, preventing fat burning. Rye contains a lectin that settles in the vascular system. Corn and buckwheat do gain weight more than other foods.

Very Beneficial: Rice Bran, Puffed Rice, Spelled, Rice Crackers, Oatmeal, Rice Flour, Rice Bran, Oat Bran.

Neutrals: White Rice, Brown Rice, Flaked Oats, Barley, Cream of Rice, Starch, Granola, Quinoa, Malta, Millet (all).

Not Advisable: Amaranth, Cassava, Rye, Pop Corn, Cream of Wheat, Wheat Germ, Corn Flour, Corn Flakes, Corn of Any Kind, Kamut, Kasha (wheat porridge), Sorghum Millet, No Wheat product, Pop Corn, Wheat Bran, Topinambur, All kinds of Corn including Jojoto or Elote, Crumbled Wheat, Buckwheat, Durum Wheat Semolina.

BREADS.

Avoid wheat, corn, buckwheat, and rye. Try the **Essene or Ezekiel** breads (in health food **stores**).

Very Beneficial: Unrefined Rice Bread, Essene Bread, Ezekiel Bread, Rice Crackers.

Neutrals: Arab Bread, High Protein Bread without Wheat, Spelled Bread, Gluten Free Bread, Rice Bread, Oat Bran Bread, Pumpernickel.

Not Advisable: Rye Bread, Wheat Bread, Soy Flour Bread, Whole Wheat Bread, Multi-Cereals, Corn Muffins, Wheat Bran Bread, Wheat Thread.

FLOURS AND PASTA.

Grain, flour and pasta options are the same as for breads and cereals. Minimize your intake of pasta and rice.

Very Beneficial: Oatmeal, Brown Rice Flour.

Neutral: Unrefined Rice, Semolina Noodles, Spinach Quinoa Noodles, White Rice and Basmati Noodles, White Flour (eventually and in a small amount the flour that is mixed with corn and rice), Graham Flour, Spelled Flour.

No Available: Rice India, Couscous, Pasta Soy Flour, rye flour, barley flour Integral Wheat Flour, Wheat Bulgur Flour, Wheat Hard, gluten, soy flour, kasha Wheat Saracen, Pasta of Artichoke.

VEGETABLES.

Very Beneficial: Garlic, Sweet Potatoes, Eggplant, Broccoli, Chinese Cabbage, Kale, Brussels Sprouts, Cauliflower, Parsnip (white carrot), Beet greens, Mustard greens, Oriental Mushroom (shiitake), Ginger, Turnips, Parsnip, Potato Little (sweet potato), Parsley, Paprika, Half Moon Bean, Beet (little), Cabbage, Brussels Sprouts, Yam, Carrots.

Neutrals: Chard, Agar, Alfalfa, Algae of all kinds, Chili peppers, Chicory, Seaweed, Celery, Pea, Pumpkin, Watercress, Bamboo shoots, Zucchini, Chestnut, Onions, Kohlrabi, Dandelion, Endive, Dill, Escalonia, Endive, Asparagus, Spinach, Chayote (shallot), Peas, Fennel, Oriental Enoki Mushroom, Abalone Mushrooms, Lettuce of All Kinds, Ocumo, Chinese Ocumo, Potato (little), Cucumber, Perifolio, Leek, Okra, Horseradish, Radicheta, Arugula, Rutabaga, Pods, Yucca (little), Zucchini.

Not Recommended: Avocado, Greek Olives, Black and Green Olives (their mold can cause allergic reactions), Acacia (gum arabic), Artichoke, Swiss Thistle, Senna leaves, Yellow and White Corn, Rhubarb, Radish, Tempe (fermented soybeans), Tofu (soy cheese), Tomato (eliminate them from your diet because they have a gluing heme lectin that irritates your stomach lining), All Aloe-Based Products (zabila), Jerusalem artichoke, Topinambur or Pataca.

FRUITS.

Very Beneficial: Blueberry, Cambur Apple Tree, Plum (all kinds), Cherries, Prunes, Guava, Fresh Figs (except prickly pear), Lechosa (papaya), Mirtillos, Blackberries, Pineapple (it has a digestive enzyme and is diuretic) , Watermelon, Grape (all).

Neutrals: Elderberries, Cocoa, Long Cambur, Coconut, Apricots (apricot), Dates, Peach, Raspberry, Strawberries, Wild Currant, Soursop, Dried Figs, Kiwi, Lime, Litchi, Lemon, Mamón, Tangerine, Mango, Apple, Melon (all kinds), Peach, Quinces, Oranges, Nectarine, Parchita (little), Raisins (raisins, raisins), Pear, Banana, Grapefruit (grapefruit), Prunas, Quinotos, Elderberry, Blackberry.

Not Advisable: Avocado, Carambola (Chinese tamarind or star fruit), Persimmon or Kaki, Prunes, Pomegranate, Prickly Pear, Rhubarb.

JUICES AND LIQUIDS.

When you get up, have a **"fluidizing cocktail"** made with 1 tablespoon of flaxseed oil, 1 tablespoon of granules (also comes in capsules) <u>of soy lecithin</u> and one cup of allowed fruit juice. Shake and drink. **This provides you with high levels of choline, serine, and ethanolamine, phospholipids that are very beneficial for type B.**

Very Beneficial : Filtered and Ozonized Water, Rice Drinks (bottle, chicha), Pineapple Juice, Cranberry Juice, Cabbage Juice, Milky Juice, Grape Juice, Carrot Juice, Green Tea, Ginseng Tea, Tea of Ginger, Mint Tea, Licorice Tea.

Neutrals: Water with Lemon (water, little lemon, little sugar), Drinking Water, Coffee (little), Beer, Celery Juice, Black Plum Juice, Damascus Juice (apricot), Apple Juice, Orange Juice, Juice Cucumber, Grapefruit Juice, Prune Juice, Apple Cider, Black Tea (little), Wines.

Not Advisable: Tomato Juice and in No Presentation, Grape Juice, Distilled Liquors, Aloe Tea (Zabila).

SPICES.

Strong herbs are good for them, while **sweet ones irritate their stomachs.**

Very Beneficial: Curry, Ginger, Parsley in General, Cayenne Pepper, Horseradish.

Neutral: Agar, Savory, Chili Peppers, Basil, Capers without Vinegar, Caraway (cumin of meadow), Seaweed and Red, Carob, Anise, Arrowroot, Saffron, Stevia Sugar (little), Cardamom, Chives, Clove, Cilantro, Cumin, Cream of Tartar, Coriander, Turmeric, Cocoa Powder, Dill, Tarragon, Maple Syrup, Rice Syrup (very little), Laurel, Yeast (little), Tangerine, Marjoram, Mint, Mustard (Without vinegar), Mustard in Powder, Nutmeg, Oregano, Paprika, Chinese Parsley, Perifolio, Paprika, Peppercorns, Licorice Root, Rosemary, Salt, Sage Powder, Tamarind, Thyme, Balsamic Vinegar (from white and red sugar-free cider).

Not Advisable: Refined Sugar, Brown Sugar, Cinnamon, Almond Extract (essence), Fructose, Pure Gelatin, Glucose, Sugar Cane Syrup, Corn Syrup, Juniper, Cornstarch, Barley Malt, Molasses, Bee Honey, Mustard with Vinegar, Ground Black and White Pepper, Soy Sauce, Vanilla.

CONDIMENTS.

Very Beneficial: None.

Neutrals: Acid Pickles (without vinegar), Sweets and Kosher, Mayonnaise (without vinegar), Mustard Sauce, Pickled Cucumbers with Dill, Worcestershire Sauce.

Not Advisable: Fruit Jellies, Ketchup And No Ketchup, Jams.

HERB INFUSIONS.

You don't get great benefits from most, and a few are harmful.

Very Beneficial: Rose Fruit, Ginseng (positive effect on the nervous system, but can act as a stimulant, so drink it in the morning), **Raspberry Leaf, Ginger, Palo Dulce** (elixir for chronic fatigue, it is antiviral and levels sugar in blood), Mint (softens the digestive tract), **Parsley, Sage.**

Neutrals: White Birch, Alfalfa, Álsine (stellar), Burdock, Cayenne, White Oak Bark, Dandelion, Dong Quai (phytoestrogens), Echinacea (stimulates the immune system), St. John's Wort, Catnip, Strawberry Leaf , Chamomile, Marjoleto, Horehound, Yarrow, Mulberry, American Elm, Orozuz Root, Elderberry, Thyme, Valerian, Verbena, Sarsaparilla.

Not Recommended: Fenugreek, Aloe (Aloe), Corn Beard, Candlemas, Skullcap, Horse's Claw, Gentian, Hops, Rhubarb, Sen, Linden, Red Clover.

DRINKS (stimulants).

This group feels best when you limit your drinks to green tea, herbal teas, water, and juices. While tea, coffee and wine do not harm them, they do not boost their performance. The **green tea** has caffeine, but also antioxidants.

Very Beneficial: Ozonated Water, Green Tea.

Neutral: Filtered drinking water, Coffee, Beer, Black Tea, White and Red Wine.

Not Advisable: Mineral Water (contains heavy minerals that agglutinate the blood), Seltz Water (sparkling water), Soft drinks of any kind, Malta, Distilled Liquors.

SUPPLEMENTS FOR TYPE B.

His diet is already rich in vitamins A, B, C and E, calcium and iron. The goal is to improve an already balanced diet, ensure insulin efficiency, strengthen viral immunity, and improve concentration and mental clarity.

Magnesium: It is the catalyst for the metabolic mechanism of type B that makes you metabolize carbohydrates more efficiently. Because you absorb calcium well, you risk throwing your calcium / magnesium levels out of balance, lowering your immunity to viruses and can lead to fatigue, depression, and nervous disorders.

Many children in this group suffer from eczema and the supplement may be beneficial to them. You can try 300-500 mg, but be aware that magnesium citrate has a laxative effect on you. It's in all the vegetables, grains, and legumes recommended for your type of diet.

Recommended Herbs / Phytochemicals: Palo dulce (glycyrrhiza glabra) treats stomach ulcers, is an antiviral agent against herpes, treats fatigue syndrome and fights hypoglycemia (1 or 2 cups of palo palo tea after lunch and dinner).

Digestive enzymes: If you are not used to eating meat, take them for a while. **Bromeliad (from pineapple)** is purchased in health food stores, they **improve retention and concentration.** The best herb is **Siberian Ginseng (Eleutherococcus senticosus) and Ginkgo Biloba which increases the micro-circulation of the brain.**

Lecithin: Blood purifier. **The fluidizing cocktail (see in juices and liquids)** of the blood is an excellent stimulant of the immune system.

FOODS THAT DEGENERATE.

- **Lentils:** They inhibit the proper assimilation of nutrients, affecting metabolic efficiency, causing hypoglycemia.

- **Sesame seed:** Affects metabolic efficiency causing hypoglycemia.

- **Corn:** Inhibits insulin efficiency, slows metabolic rate, causes hypoglycemia.

- **Buckwheat:** Inhibits digestion affects metabolic efficiency causing hypoglycemia.

- **Wheat:** It slows down the digestive and metabolic processes, causing food to be stored as fat, and not burning as energy, inhibits insulin efficiency.

FOODS THAT REGENERATE.

- **Green leafy vegetables:** They promote metabolic efficiency.

- **Meat:** Promotes metabolic efficiency.

- **Eggs-dairy products:** Promote low-fat metabolic efficiency.

- **Liver:** Promotes metabolic efficiency.

OTHER RECOMMENDATIONS...

- **Healthy Longevity Book... How to Live 100 Years Appearing Much Less.**
- **The Cookbook... Personalized According to your Blood Group.**
- **Certified Courses for Professionals and Aspiring Therapists.**

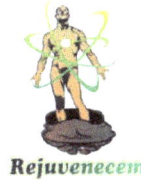

The House of Children Foundation...
We recommend the **"BOOK TO HEALTHY LONGEVITY GROUP B DIABETIC".**
The goal... Live 100 years Appearing much less... Because if you can... **Bring:**

- How to eat and Rejuvenate according to your Blood Group.
- Special Exercises to Increase Health.
- Golden Tips that will make you lead a Much Better Life.
- How to eat after 45.
- How to Regenerate Metabolism.

- How to clean the liver, bile ducts, colon and kidneys.

- Alkalinity Life - Acids Death.

- How Emotional Conflicts Kill.

- Why We Age and How to Rejuvenate (2,023)...

- Local and Systemic Mushroom Cleaning

- 9 Foods to Have More Intense Intimate Relationships.

- The 12 Best Nutrients for Life Extension.

THE KITCHEN RECIPE FOR DIABETIC GROUP B...

It is personalized according to your blood group, where you can prepare delicacies that will rejuvenate you and in a simple way.... Bring:

- How to Prepare the Best Sauces.

- How to Prepare the Best Mayonnaise.

- Preparation of Smoked Bones at home.

- Prepare the best Chimichurri or Guasacaca that you have ever eaten.

- Italian Sea Salt, For Salads, Meats, Seafood, Fish and Poultry.

➤ Broths for: Meat, Seafood, Chicken, Chicken, Fish.

➤ Unrivaled Starters, Salads, Soups, Creams and Main Dishes.

➤ Yyyy of course the best Christmas dishes.

And remember that your Blessing will Help Many Needy here at La Casa De DIOS Foundation and where we will be praying for your seed to be paid in health for you and you're Family.

The Cookbook will find it at this link. www.fundaciondeterapeutas.com

COURSES.

✚ Certified Courses for Professionals and Aspiring Therapists.

Sai-Medic Institute for Scientific Research.
Attacking the Cause. Effects Disappear.
Center for Alternatives
Scientific Health Research.

Rejuveneceme

With more than 45 years of experience in hundreds of thousands of patients and using the latest advances in science, we will indicate you with simple, but powerful recommendations, how to treat the problems that afflict humanity in such a fast and palpable way, that you will believe. Find out why we get sick and age. How to quickly rejuvenate and heal...

Ownership of the Course Certified by the Institute will be delivered.

Professional Courses.

COURSE Chosen.

1- Neuro Advanced Acupuncture. Energy Systems.

2- Food to have more intense relationships.

3- How to Regenerate According to the Blood Group.

4- How to Rejuvenate.

5- Cancer If Cured.

6- Obesity ... Lose Weight Immediately.

7- How to cure type 2 diabetes in a short time.

"May GOD be our Strength"

CURRICULUM VITAE

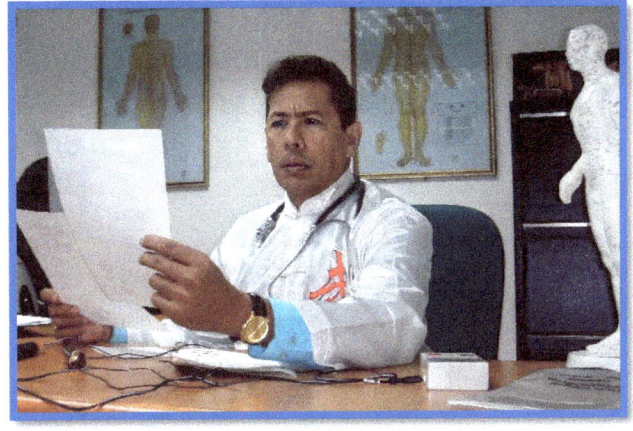

Name: M. A Ramoni

Web: fundaciondeterapeutas.com

Professional Studies:

- ENAHO (National School of Acupuncture and Homeopathy). Years 1983 to 1989.

- Studies at the Venezuelan School of Psychotronic Society. 1989 Caracas Venezuela.

- Studies of the Food Yin Yang Macrobiotic knowledge of Dr. Sakurazawa Nyoiti of Japanese origin, through Professor Omar Viera.

- Korean Acupuncture (Koryo Sooji Chim Acupuncture Mano koryo) from Master Dr. Yoo Tae W received with a Three Level program at the National School of Acupuncture and Homeopathy through Dr. Omar Viera.

➤ Studies of Dr. José Luís Padilla Corral, director of the School of MT Ch. "Neijing" Spain.

➤ Regression hypnosis INME Institute (Experimental Meta-gnomic Institute).

➤ Didactic Homeosineatry. From the Bathem Bathen school.

➤ Iridology. International Federation of Iris Diagnosis. From the Federation of Dr. Omar Viera.

➤ Maxilo-Facial anti-wrinkle treatment through the dermatron and electo-acupuncture. 2009 (I continue).

➤ Food According to the Blood Group. Research researcher James and Peter D'adamo. 2008. (I continue).

➤ Rejuvenation through the lengthening of the telomeres. 2010 (I continue).

➤ Alkalinity and acidity of cells in the development of diseases. 2010 (I continue).

➤ Master in Energy Systems.

- Master in Anesthesia by Electro Acupuncture.
- Master in Pain Therapies.
- Master in Iridology (Diagnosis by Iris).
- Neuropsychology. The New Medicine of the Future. Dr Hamer Germany.

JOBS:

- President and founder of the Scientific Research Institute of Alternative Health Medicines SAID-MEDIC.
- Director of the Said-Medic La Maracaya Medical Center clinic from 1988 to 1992.
- Director of the Said-Medic Lourdes Medical Center clinic from 1993 to 1995.
- Director of the Said-Medic Medical Center clinic Dungeon from the year 1996 to the year 2,000.
- Professor in courses for Doctors and Para-Doctors in Homeopathy - Acupuncture 1st Level - 2nd Level - 3rd Level and Energy Systems.

➤ Director of the Las Acacias Said-Medic Medical Center clinic from the year 2010 to the year 2012.

➤ Director of the Said-Medic Palmarito Medical Center clinic from year 2013 to year 2017.

➤ Director of the Said-Medic Street Páez Medical Center clinic from 2.017 to 2.023.

➤ Professor, Lecturer, International Bioenergetics Seminary - Neuro Acupuncture - Food according to the Blood Group - Why we age and how to rejuvenate - Main diseases, Neuro Psychology, among others.

WRITER OF MEDICINE BOOKS:

1- Rejuvenate, lose weight, be strong and healthy.

2- Food According to Blood Group "O".

3- Blood Group Healthy Longevity Guide A.

4- Blood Group Healthy Longevity Guide A Diabetic.

5- Blood Group Healthy Longevity Guide AB.

6- Blood Group Healthy Longevity Guide Ab Diabetic.

7- Blood Group Healthy Longevity Guide B.

8- Blood Group Healthy Longevity Guide B Diabetic.

9- Blood Group Healthy Longevity Guide O.

10- Blood Group Healthy Longevity Guide O Diabetic.

11- Food According to Blood Group "A"

12- Food According to Blood Group "B"

13- Food According to the Blood Group "AB"

14- Food According to the Diabetic Blood Group "O"

15- Food According to the Diabetic Blood Group "A"

16- Food According to the Diabetic Blood Group "B"

17- Food According to the Diabetic Blood Group "AB"

18- Blood Group Cookery Recipe "O".

19- Blood Group Cookbook "A"

20- Blood Group Cookbook "B"

21- Blood Group Cookbook "AB"

22- Cooking Recipe Group Diabetic Blood "O"

23- Cooking Recipe Group Diabetic Blood "A"

24- Cooking Recipe Diabetic Blood Group "B"

25- **<u>Cooking Recipe</u>** Diabetic Blood Group "AB"

26- Cancer if cured ... Educate, Alkalize and Balance.

27- Slimy Blood Syndrome ... The Cause of All Diseases.

28- How to Cure the Prostate.

29- Free yourself from Arthritis.

30- Farewell to Rheumatism.

31- Obesity ... Lose Weight Immediately and never Gain Fat again.

32- Alkalinity Life - Acidity Death.

33- Diabetes if Cured.

34- Say Goodbye to Hypertension.

35- Constipation ... Dark Future.

36- Convert your Pain into Well-being ... Legs, Lumbago, Sciatica, Spine and Cervical, among others.

37- Regenerate yourself from ACV

38- How to Eliminate Kidney and Gallstones.

39- Liver, Bile Duct, Gallbladder and colon cleansing

40- Cure Gastritis and Gastro Esophageal Reflux.

41- Say goodbye to asthma.

42- Because we grow old.

43- Tell me your Conflict ... And I will tell you that you suffer.

OTHER BOOKS:

1- CROSS POETRY. (Poetry, Updating).

2- 7 MINUTES. (Thriller, Updating).

PROFESSIONAL ASSOCIATIONS:

- Member of the WHO (World health organization number 0023 for Latin America, in alternative health medicines, through ENAHO).

- Member of the International Acupunture Association.

- College of Homeopaths and Natural Alternative Medicine Sciences.

- Venezuelan Federation of Natural Alternative Medicines N° 0024V as well as Member of the International Centers of Homeopathy and

Acupuncture of: CHCMANV N° CHV002-A - INCIHOVE N° 00020 AVA 051-V.

SPECIALTIES.

1- Diagnostic Specialist.

2- Cancer if cured.

3- Neuropathies.

4- Column.

5- Cervical.

6- Some (pain) of any kind.

7- Type 2 and 3 diabetes If it is cured.

8- Type 1 diabetes (Mellitus) exponentially improves the quality of life.

9- Arthritis.

10- Rheumatism.

11- Obesity.

12- Diseases without Cause Diagnosis.

13- Migraine, Headache.

14- Digestive System.

15- ACV

16- Body, Mental and Dynamic Rejuvenation.

17- Asthma.

18- Allergies.

19- Lupus.

20- Emotional Conflicts.

21- Traumas.

22- Renal Deficiency.

23- Neurological Senile dementia, Parkinson's, Alzheimer's, Huntington.

24- Seizures.

25- Hypertension ... Among many others.

"If we eliminate the cause ... the effects are eliminated."

"The Course that Rules Nature ...
It is the Artistic Expression of *GOD*."

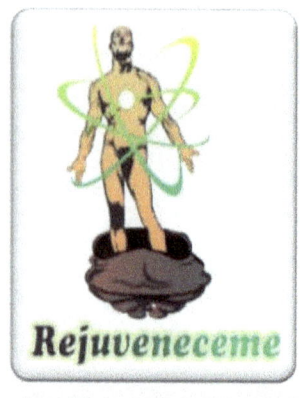

> Now, reread one by one the important topics that you will find in the Healthy Longevity Guide, in relation to the new culture of rejuvenation - healing and get rid of once and forever, that damaged state that so much hinders a body healthy.

www.fundaciondeterapeutas.com   **2.023.**

DEDICATION...

I want to dedicate this and all the good things I have done in this world to the one who deserves it the most and that is my Heavenly Father.

Jehovah of Hosts...

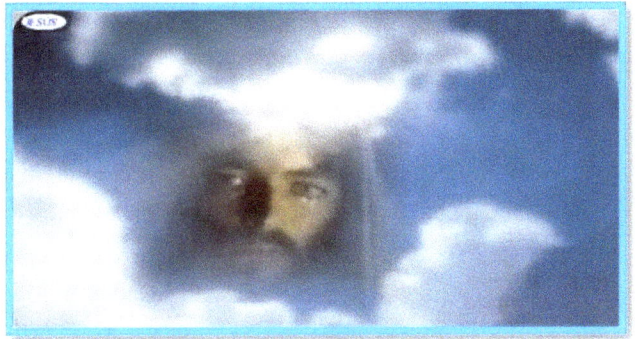

Thank you, I love you very much and... In the name of **GOD** ...I wish you the best...

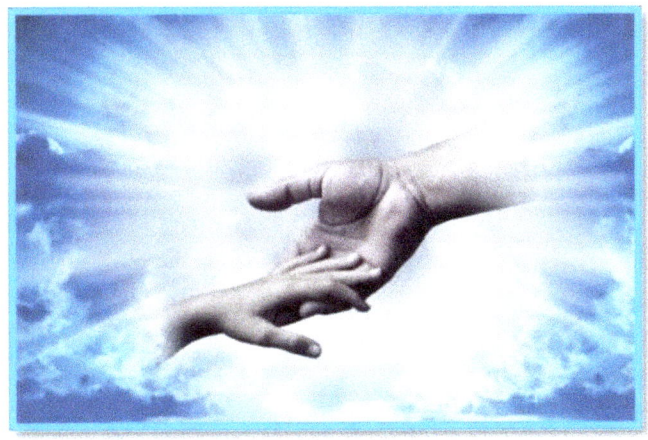

So... Never forget, that when science says... I can't anymore... **GOD** says... I start...

www.ingramcontent.com/pod-product-compliance
Lightning Source LLC
Chambersburg PA
CBHW072304170526
45158CB00003BA/1188